The Ketogenic Diet

How to use Ketosis to Lose Weight, Increase Mental Focus, & Feel Truly Alive!

By Oliver Ryan

SCHOFIELD PUBLISHING HOUSE

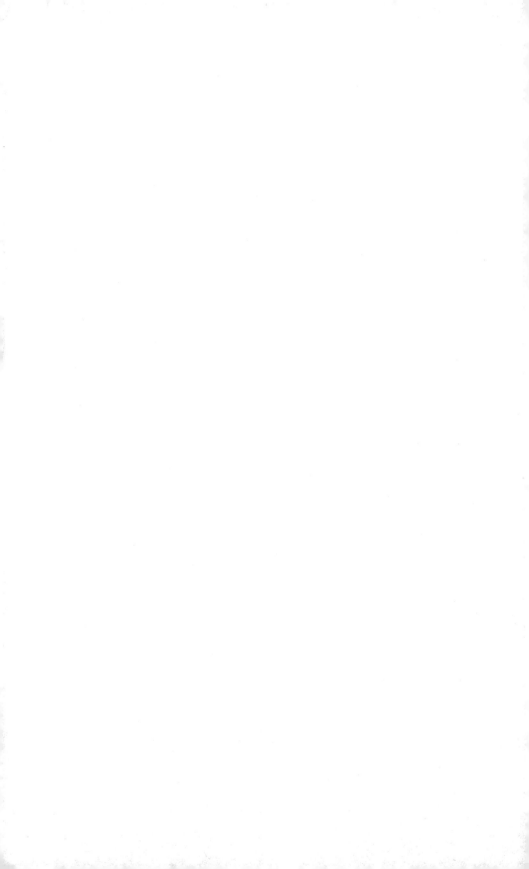

TABLE OF CONTENTS

Introduction

I want to thank you and congratulate you for purchasing the book, "Ketogenic Diet: How to use Ketosis to Lose Weight, Increase Mental Focus, & Feel Truly Alive."

You are on your way to beginning a revolutionary journey to losing weight, improving your health, and changing your lifestyle. The ketogenic diet is a proven way to achieve these easily without having to sacrifice your palate, or worse, go hungry. The problem with most diets is that they require a drastic change in eating patterns, a significant decrease in caloric intake, and a reduction in the palatability of the new regimen. That is why very few people fare well in the various diets, so much so that the average American goes on a diet to lose weight about ten times in a lifetime, and he almost always ultimately fails.

The ketogenic diet is not a fad diet, and has actually been around for decades. Over the past forty years, high-fat diets have been proven to be successful in weight loss and health improvement, and have been marketed, with staggering success, by a few. In addition, almost a hundred years ago, high fat diets were actually used to treat epilepsy in small children, a condition that is difficult to control. This just shows that even then, dietary fat was instrumental in improving neural function in humans.

The ketogenic diet has been steadily winning devotees and fans because of a huge number of successful dieters. There are also many dieticians and health professionals all over the world who have gone public touting the benefits of the diet. These same professionals have also publicly assailed the so-called "ideal" and balanced diets promoted by national and international medical associations and governments. Enlightened high-fat diet proponents now dismiss these diets as wrong and downright dangerous.

In this book, we will elevate dietary fat to its deserved pedestal, and show that it is not only recommended, but required, for a life of optimal health and vitality.

I encourage you to start this exciting journey to a longer, more vibrant lifestyle.

Thank you again for purchasing this book. I hope you enjoy it!

Chapter One
Fat Becomes a Bad Word

Dietary fat has been pretty much demonized since U.S. and international health authorities began to give recommendations on what people should, or shouldn't, eat. They conjured up a so-called "balanced diet" that is actually biased in favor of carbohydrate intake (because of the influence of the agricultural sector), at the expense of the macronutrient fat, which became the code word for bad health and irresponsible nutrition. Fat became quickly linked to coronary disease, weight gain, increase in cholesterol levels, and other associated health problems.

So-called dietary "experts" began calling for people to limit their daily intake of fat to as little as 10% of their total caloric intake, while recommending that the percentage share of carbohydrates in all its forms, be increased to as much as 70%. These recommendations, far from improving the health of Americans, have actually led to higher obesity rates, an increase in the incidence of heart disease, and a rise in metabolic disease cases, especially diabetes. With the rise of these health problems, the prescription for reducing fat intake was apparently an ill-conceived one, reflecting a disastrous lack of understanding of how the human body was designed, and where it is supposed to obtain energy for fuel.

In the Dietary Guidelines for America issued by the U.S. Department of Agriculture 2015-2020 Edition, the diagram, "My Plate" shows five food groups that they recommend to be part of the daily diet: fruits, grains, vegetables, protein, and dairy. There is nothing in diagram that suggests that fat should be included in the diet. The government suggests that at least three-fifths of a person's caloric intake be comprised of three categories -- fruits, grains, and vegetable -- which collectively include mostly carbohydrates. Fats are included in a mention of oils, with the guide stating that "Oils are fats that are liquid at room temperature, like the vegetable oils used in cooking. Oils come from many different plants and from fish. Oils are NOT (emphasis ours) a food group, but they provide essential nutrients."

In the government guidelines, the oils are instead included in food "patterns," instead of being a major food group. Fat as a dietary component is practically excluded from the nutrition discussion on a government level!

The problem is, relegating dietary fat to the role of evil macronutrient ignores the metabolic processes that the human body have been operating on for four million years or so. For well over 99.9% of their chronological existence, human beings, hunting animals for their main source of food, ingested plenty of animal fat for their body's energy needs. The archaeological record shows that our prehistoric ancestors were lean, muscular, and fit as a result of their diet.

Their average life spans were shortened by over half of today's Homo sapiens not because of dietary choices but because of early deaths in childhood and adolescence, the absence of drugs, and the harsh conditions of the time. For about 3,990,000 years, the human being was molded and shaped by his diet, which seemed to have given them health, and along with strenuous activity, that chiseled, "surfer dude" look. Ingesting zero processed carbohydrates and eating mostly animal fat did our prehistoric ancestors a lot of good. Prehistoric man proved that carbohydrates are not essential nutrients. Today, in fact, there are groups of people, such as the Masai tribe of Africa, and the Inuit of Alaska, who thrive on these high-fat, prehistoric diets, and survive without carbohydrates for extended periods of time without any ill effects on their well-being, and health. This is lost on an overwhelming majority of the rest of the human race, which continue on the unhealthy road of high-carbohydrate diets.

It was only about 10,000 years ago that mankind stopped its hunter-gatherer ways, and with that, they discovered agriculture and its malevolent products: processed carbohydrates, especially wheat, sugar, and flour. When prehistoric man stopped moving around, and began to settle into permanent living spaces, he found ways to grow these new types of food, such as grains, and add them to their stores to feed the rapidly increasing populations. Humans also found ways to process and "refine" them, so that they could be stored for future use, especially during droughts and winters, and for when the occasional famine struck. Eventually, these storage methods led to processes that dehydrated, and preserved them, especially grains.

To make food more palatable and interesting, humans also developed countless forms and formulations of sweeteners and sugars to improve the taste of food. But our bodies reacted rather adversely to these "new" dietary inputs. Humans started becoming fatter and unhealthier, partly because of lifestyle, and partly because human bodies were not designed to ingest these types of carbohydrates. Human metabolic processes were meant to process small amounts of naturally-occurring carbohydrates, and turn them to glucose for quick use and expenditure. The extra glucose in the bloodstream usually ends up in muscle tissue as glycogen, eventually becoming fat, and adding to the body's fat stores.

While modern medicine and better information has helped humanity to prolong life spans through better drugs and treatment, humans now get fatter, and contract diabetes and heart disease at a much earlier age than hundreds of years ago. Today's obese American is the culmination of this so-called agricultural "progress" – continually struggling to get slender and healthy as they consume higher and higher levels of carbohydrates. Worse, because of public misinformation, today's Homo sapiens are struggling to solve the diet problem.

To lose weight and be fit, our bodies need to revert to eating much less carbohydrates. This is where ketosis and the ketogenic diet come in.

Chapter Two
The Chemistry Of Life – Understanding Ketosis

The biochemical processes involved in the human body getting its fuel and energy supply are complex. However, it is important to understand the basics of such processes on a cellular level in order to appreciate the significance of ketosis, and the ketogenic diet.

To understand the metabolic processes better, it is useful to liken the human body to a car with an internal combustion engine - one that requires the correct type of fuel to run. Like an automobile, the human body requires fuel to make it run and perform at peak levels. While internal combustion engines run on petroleum, the human body "runs" on food.

Digestion and metabolism transform the food that we eat into the fuel that allows the body to function -- and function properly. However, unlike a car which does not need fuel when its engine is turned off, the human body still needs to use and process fuel even while it is at rest, or at a dormant state. The human body even needs to utilize fuel even when it is asleep: human hearts still pump, lungs still process the air you breathe, digestive processes still take place, and so on. The human body needs a constant supply of fuel every second of every day, and diet provides the fuel.

To obtain this fuel from their diet, humans eat three basic types of food that serve different roles for the nourishment and maintenance of the human body: proteins, carbohydrates, and fats. These three dietary nutrients are digested, metabolized, and serve the body in different, and specific ways.

Food is converted to fuel through the process of metabolism, which starts from the time that we put the food in our mouth and chew it until it is broken down, and converted into the nutrients that fuel our body's needs. There are three basic "macronutrients" that have different features as fuel and energy sources.

Proteins

These come from lean meats, poultry, seafood, dairy products, nuts, grains and beans. Proteins are broken down into amino acids, and its primary purpose is to facilitate tissue growth and repair. It is the body's least favorite source of energy, and for a good reason – the body needs proteins to maintain, and create body tissue and membranes.

Protein synthesis releases amino acids (the building blocks of proteins), which are moved into muscle cells and incorporated into larger proteins. However, if protein is the only available food, the body metabolizes it into other amino acids; it can even be converted into sugars for energy purposes. If we eat just protein to satisfy the body's energy needs, the body will have less of it to strengthen muscle and tissue, leading to muscle loss, as muscle tissue wastes away. This can lead to serious nutritional deficiencies, and even death.

Because of this, protein is the least desirable macro-nutrient for energy purposes. In a 150-pound human body, which is the average, with around 20% of body fat, there is approximately thirteen pounds of muscle protein available for fuel use, most of it to be used for vital tissue growth, replacement, and repair.

Carbohydrates

We will spend a lot more time discussing carbohydrates, because we first need to understand that they are the "culprit" behind obesity and metabolic diseases – NOT fat, and second, carbs are what the human body seeks out first when it is starving for fuel. The body utilizes them, as its first and quickest source of energy. Carbs are the most accessible, cheapest and widely available source of body fuel today. While this sounds well and good (why use fat at all?), it pays to understand how carbohydrates are broken down, used, and in the next chapter, why ingesting a lot is not a good idea.

As mentioned in Chapter 1, dietary carbohydrates are the most readily available food, partly due to organized agriculture. Consider the following list:

Grains (Rice and wheat, also made into bread)

Fruits (Most contain fructose)

Milk (Most contain galactose and lactose)

Vegetables (Most contain maltose), potatoes, and other starches

Table sugar, and Splenda (Sucrose)

Candy and syrup

Beans and legumes

Carbohydrates can also be classified as either simple or complex, depending on a carbohydrate's chemical structure of the food, and how easily and/or quickly the sugar in the food is processed and absorbed. Simple carbohydrates have one or two sugar molecules. These carbohydrates have a high glycemic index, which means that they are more easily convertible to glucose in the bloodstream. Examples of these carbohydrates are highly "processed" foods", like refined sugar, high fructose corn syrup, white rice, and white bread.

On the other hand, complex carbohydrates are compounds with three or more molecules. These carbohydrates have a low glycemic index, which means that they are less easily convertible to glucose in tine bloodstream. Examples of complex carbohydrates are peanuts, lentils, peas, starchy foods like potatoes and yams, and cereals and whole-grain bread products. Nutritionists love complex carbohydrates because most of them contain fiber, which aids digestion and gives a feeling of "fullness." They also supposedly contain chemicals that induce sleep, and help establish sleeping patterns. Carbohydrates are a fast-acting source of energy for the body, but they do not do a lot to provide a feeling of satiation or fullness: Even carbohydrates that are supposedly loaded with fiber are far less filling than protein or fat.

One of nature's main purposes for "creating" carbohydrates was to somehow transfer the sun's energy to human metabolism. Photosynthesis, or the process where organisms, especially green plants, transform the light energy into chemical energy, is the fundamental process that maintains life on Earth – providing fuel and energy to the flora, and indirectly, to animals.

Plants convert this energy into its structural components, and almost all organisms derive protein, directly or indirectly, from the organic compounds formed within plants during photosynthesis. The stored energy in these compounds is essential for fuel, growth, cell repair, reproduction, movement, and other vital functions.

When carbohydrates are ingested, they are converted into blood glucose through the process of hydrolysis, and absorbed through the small intestines and enter the bloodstream, which causes blood glucose levels to rise. This process of making and transporting glucose triggers a very important hormonal action: the pancreas makes insulin, a peptide that helps bring the sugar go to the cells so that they can use it as energy. This metabolic process can go haywire when too much carbohydrate is ingested, as we will see in the next section.

When there is more glucose in the bloodstream, the pancreas secretes more insulin. This triggers excess glucose in the blood to be moved to other tissues, especially muscles, and then stored in the form of glycogen. Excess glycogen is then pushed into fat cells for storage, adding to whatever fat stores are already present. If there's enough glucose in the body, it is the preferred fuel for most tissues, but any excess amount is embedded into muscle tissue, leading to additional, unneeded fat layers.

In an average 150-pound human, there is very little carbohydrate stores available for fuel use, so in extreme cases of caloric deprivation, the body has no carbohydrate stores to provide sustenance for the body. Carbohydrate fuel needs constant re-supply to give the human body a feeling of being satiated, or "fullness." It is therefore, a very inefficient, and wasteful use of dietary calories. If humans need to use carbohydrates as their only source of fuel, they need to constantly be eating carbohydrates, round the clock!

Prehistoric man did not have much need for the sun-infused carbohydrates, because they were exposed to the sun much more than modern man is today. Almost all of their activity, especially travelling and hunting, were done while being exposed to the sun's rays. Humans however, began producing processed carbohydrates way in excess of the normal levels required. When these additional processed carbohydrates somehow crept into humanity's diet, and became one of its major food sources, human beings began to, in effect, consume unneeded nutrients. This redundancy in nutrition has led to a variety of illnesses prevalent today.

Fat

Dietary fat comes from land animals, poultry, seafood, and secondary sources, such as oils derived from vegetables, seeds, and other animal fat. Unlike proteins and carbohydrates, the human body can store almost an unlimited supply of calories as body fat, for fuel purposes. For our average 150-pound individual, this means having 80,000 calories worth of stored fat in his adipose tissue. Also, of the three major dietary sources—protein, carbohydrates, and fat—fat contains the most calories per gram, with about 9 calories per gram, while protein and carbohydrates have 4 calories per gram. Fat storage of this amount theoretically contains enough energy to allow someone to walk around 800 miles, before the body has to tap into extra fuel.

This is precisely the reason that prehistoric man could survive for days without any food, and why people who go on hunger strikes, for example, do not need to eat anything for several days, since the body simply uses the fat stores that it already has. During a period of total starvation, the body uses just up to 2,000 calories per day, so with 80,000 calories of stored fat - a human being can go for over 40 days without food, before the body starts to break down.

Ketosis

A main objective of the ketogenic diet is to ensure that the human body doesn't have enough dietary carbohydrates, which we have shown is the most inefficient source of body fuel, to burn for energy. The greatest rates of fat oxidation or use, will occur under conditions when carbohydrates are restricted and even eliminated, and when fat consumption is increased.

In a high-fat, very low-carbohydrate diet, the body will burn fat, instead of carbohydrates, and as part of this process, it will make ketones. Ketones are made in the liver from fatty acids, generated from the breakdown of fats. Ketones are formed almost as a defensive action by the body: when it "senses" that there is not enough sugar or glucose to provide for the body's energy needs, it immediately creates this alternative fuel source.

When dietary carbohydrates are suddenly taken away from the diet, the pancreas secretes less insulin, while more fatty acids are then released from fat cells, which leads to more of these fats being burned up in our liver. This increased burning of fatty acids in the liver eventually causes ketone bodies to be produced, and induces ketosis, a new metabolic state. Other hormones are likewise affected, and these transfer ketone bodies, instead of carbohydrates, to body tissues. The majority of calories burned up by the human body will now come from this fat breakdown.

When the human body is in a state of ketosis, it creates a "glucose sparing" effect. In this condition, the skeletal muscles first burn the fatty acids which "spare" glucose for the brain to use. Second, when the body has already adapted to ketosis after the first two weeks or so, the brain switches to utilizing ketone bodies for most of its fuel needs, so glucose is no longer required.

A tiny percentage of carbohydrate usage will remain, from the obligatory usage of glucose by certain tissues.

Chapter Three
The (Bad) Effects of Carbohydrate Overconsumption

In Chapter 1, we pointed out that dietary fat has been pretty much demonized. Conversely, carbohydrates, cheap and widely available as they are, have been elevated to the point that governments suggest that 60% of a person' caloric intake should come from them. Making carbohydrates the main component of a diet, however, is harmful, and can cause the body serious harm. "Modern" diseases such as heart disease and diabetes coincided with the widespread use of processed and refined carbohydrates in human beings' diet. The destructive effects of carbohydrates are manifested in two main health afflictions: Those arising from weight gain, and those from the disruption of metabolic processes, especially that of the pancreas.

Weight gain, unneeded increase in fat levels, and heart disease

We have shown how excess carbohydrates produce excess glycogen that can be pushed into fat cells for storage. These excess carbs are usually simple carbohydrates – the kind that is easier to break down as a nutrient, and shows up faster as unneeded glycogen in tissues.

The excess fat is added to the fat stores' already existing as adipose tissue. The accumulation of excess fat, or the inability of the body to use up already existing fat stores, leads to weight gain, and the breaking off of some of these cells can clog arteries, and cause blood circulation problems. Consumption of high levels of simple carbohydrates also increases inflammation of the arteries, causing their weakness, and leading to blood vessel diseases. It also causes an increase in Low Density Lipoprotein, or "LDL," also called "Bad cholesterol,' as the blood carries cholesterol to various tissues in the body.

Diabetes

In one of the key metabolic processes to regulate carbohydrates, the pancreas makes and secretes insulin. Insulin is produced in response to increases in blood glucose. It is a storage hormone, and is used by the body to move nutrients out of the bloodstream and into target tissues and cells so that the body can obtain energy from sugars eaten.

When carbohydrates are consumed, insulin moves glucose to the muscles to be stored as glycogen or carbohydrate fuel. A primary role of insulin is to also keep blood glucose within a certain range. However, when blood glucose levels rise to a point outside this range, insulin is released to the bloodstream to stabilize blood glucose levels. The greatest increase in blood glucose levels (and the greatest increase in insulin) occurs from the consumption of dietary carbohydrates.

When the body produces too much glucose arising from the consumption of too many carbohydrates, the pancreas ultimately is overwhelmed, and it cannot produce enough insulin to process the glucose. This inability to produce insulin indicates a pathological state called diabetes, specifically, Type I diabetes. Without insulin, glucose cannot enter the cells, and the sugar remains in the bloodstream, accumulating to abnormal levels, and the cells start to starve. A person with type 1 diabetes needs to take insulin, usually through injections or orally, to allow glucose to enter into the cells.

The Ketogenic diet can possibly help those with Type II diabetes, where the body is unable able to use insulin the right way, also called insulin resistance. Type 2 Diabetes can be prevented or delayed with a healthy lifestyle, including maintaining a healthy weight, eating sensibly, exercising regularly, and of course, going on the ketogenic diet.

Chapter Four
Advantages of the Ketogenic Diet -
The Brain is King

Benefits to the Neurological System and the Brain

Most people who think of the ketogenic diet automatically relate it to weight loss and a more slender figure. In fact, these benefits are more than enough for most people to go on the diet. There is a growing body of research and experimentation, however, that suggests that the more important advantage brought about by ketosis in the ketogenic diet may be the therapeutic value that it adds to brain health and brain function.

Brain health shows significant improvement under the Ketogenic diet. During ketosis, it has been shown that the brain can derive up to ¾ of its energy requirement from ketones. In fact, the body, including the brain, can adjust to using ketones, if glucose is not available, and may be the "preferred" fuel of many tissues. In the first three weeks of the Ketogenic diet, most tissues will meet their energy requirements, not from glucose, but all of non-protein fuel will be provided by ketones, and the breakdown of free fatty acids. Brain tissue is the most important of these, because the brain controls most, if not all, the other systemic functions of the human body. The neurological benefits of the ketogenic diet can be significant.

Improved Focus and Mental Clarity

For the brain, exposure to too much glucose can result in neurotoxicity, or the exposure of the nervous system to toxic substances. Many mental issues, such as brain fog and problems with memory, are caused by this condition. In the ketogenic diet, the reduction of the supply of glucose diminishes the levels of toxicity in the body as brain starts to use ketones as fuel. Possible results include ability to think more clearly, better focus, and better memory recall.

Epilepsy

In Chapter 1, we mentioned how high-fat diets and ketosis were used as formal treatments for curing this disease in children in the 1920's. if available. Many other studies have since been made, that attempt to shed light on the positive effects of high-fat diets, and specifically, the process of ketosis, on all human beings, including adults. In fact, as recently as June 2013, an issue of the European Journal of Clinical Nutrition maintained that the main beneficiaries for a high-fat diet are those afflicted with epilepsy.

Note that the above conditions are serious, some having grim prognoses, so a decision to start a formal, medical ketogenic diet should not be taken lightly. If someone, especially a child, is affected by one of these disorders, consulting with an experienced medical doctor, or trained nutrition professional should be made before beginning a ketogenic diet. A medical ketogenic diet should never be started without professional medical consultation.

Parkinson 's disease

Parkinson's disease is part of a class of disorders that affect the body's motor systems, with the onset coming at between the ages of 50 and 65. About one percent of people in that age population are affected with the disorder. In Parkinson's disease, the dopamine-producing cells in the brain are apparently destroyed, and the production of the neurotransmitter dopamine, which controls muscular movement, declines. The symptoms of Parkinson's disease, which include shaking, tremor, sluggish movement, stiffness, and trouble balancing, show up after 60 to 80 percent of the dopamine-producing cells in the brain are destroyed. While it is not exactly clear how a ketogenic diet alleviates the symptoms of Parkinson's disease, it is highly possible that ketones, which have an anti-inflammatory effect on the brain, may be able to mend damaged neurons. The ketones may also possibly have the capability to bypass the area in the brain that is damaged, and bring much-needed energy to other areas in the brain.

Amyotrophic Lateral Sclerosis (ALS, or Lou Gehrig 's disease)

ALS is a progressive neuro-degenerative disorder that attacks the nerve cells in the brain and the spinal cord. ALS specifically affects the motor neurons, which control voluntary muscle movement. When motor neurons die, they are no longer able to send nerve signals to the muscle fibers leading to slurred speech, difficulty swallowing, muscle weakness, and almost instantly fatal breathing. In ALS, most of the muscles begin to waste away, and the person affected becomes weaker and weaker. The exact cause of ALS is unknown, and there is no known cure for the disease. However, studies on mice and other animals show that those in a ketogenic diet experienced a greater decrease in symptoms than those who weren't.

Further Benefits

Weight and fat loss

Aside from reversing the effects of, or preventing symptoms of diabetes, the ketogenic diet will almost certainly lead to significant weight loss because it reduces excess fat stores. One major reason, especially in the first couple of weeks on the diet, is that the body lowers insulin levels, which causes the kidneys to begin to shed excess sodium, causing rapid water weight loss.

A welcome side effect of the ketogenic diet is that ketone bodies dampen the appetite, because, as the body burns up the energy from fat cells, there is not as much need to ingest food through the mouth. Many followers of the Ketogenic diet, in fact notice that they actually forget to eat at times. Low-carb diets are very effective at reducing harmful abdominal fat. Apparently, it is not only the fat loss that matters, but where the fat loss occurs. It seems that a greater proportion of fat loss comes from the abdominal cavity, where fat accumulation is greatest, and known to cause serious metabolic problems.

Decrease in cholesterol, blood pressure, and better heart health

There is a marked decrease in triglycerides, fat cells, and an increase in "good cholesterol" - High Density Lipoprotein, for those going on the ketogenic diet. HDL transports cholesterol from the various tissues to the liver, and it is either broken up or excreted, and taken away from the heart. The above conditions indicate that Ketogenic diets seem to be an effective way to reduce blood pressure, many common diseases, and consequently, to help prolong life.

Cancer

The "Warburg effect" is a theory that says that cancer is caused by cancerous cells taking up large amounts of energy in the form of glucose, and converting it to lactate to produce energy. Cancer cells feed on glucose, but unlike heart, muscle, and brain cells, which can adapt to obtaining energy from ketones, tumor cells may not be able to get enough energy from ketones. As a result, it is possible that following a ketogenic diet may starve certain cancer cells of the glucose they need to survive, leading to their destruction. This theory has been tested on occasion, and the results show some positive results.

Mitochondrial Disorders

Mitochondria are organelles found in large numbers in most human cells, where the important biochemical processes of cellular respiration and energy production occur. They are also known as the energy powerhouses of the human body. The mitochondria convert the nutrients from our diet into adenosine triphosphate, or ATP, which provides the energy to all of your cells.

When mitochondria become dysfunctional, the cells are denied the energy they need. Because the brain, muscles, heart, nervous system, and eyes demand the most energy, their cells are often the most significantly affected with a mitochondrial disorder. The disruption of these body systems causes learning and intellectual disabilities, muscle weakness, hearing and visual impairment, respiratory disorders, and even seizures. There is no cure for mitochondrial disorders, so their treatment focuses on alleviating its symptoms and improving the quality of life of the sufferer.

Proper diet is often the first stage of therapy for these disorders, where seizures are a common symptom. A high-fat, ketogenic diet, can be part of the treatment plan.

Increased Energy

When the body breaks down fat instead of carbohydrates, more energy is produced for each ounce of fat used, leaving the ketogenic dieter with a feeling of heightened alertness and increased energy.

Chapter Five
Myths about the Ketogenic Diet

Despite the growing evidence that ketogenic diets can greatly improve a person's health and well-being, there are still more detractors than are supporters who maintain that a high-fat diet is an unhealthy nutrition option. Below are the more common arguments against the ketogenic diet:

Myth#1: Carbohydrates are an essential nutrient for good health.

Many nutrition professionals are overly concerned about a condition called hypoglycemia, or the lack of glucose in the bloodstream, and believe that carbohydrates are necessary to provide brain fuel. It is an antiquated way of thinking, and one that is not scientifically sound. The human body's metabolism which was developed in the course of four million years has proven that there are essential nutrients that the body itself cannot manufacture, and they have to be obtained through external food sources. At the end of Chapter 2, we showed how the body adapts to using ketone bodies for nourishing various tissues of the body, especially, the brain. When necessary, the body can also make glucose from the protein found in food. Our prehistoric ancestors have proven that there are essential proteins to build tissue, and essential fatty acids to provide fuel, but there is nothing in man's history that indicates that there is such a thing as essential carbohydrates.

Myth#2: Eating a low-carbohydrate diet can lead to vitamin deficiencies, especially that of Vitamin C, which comes from carbohydrate-rich sugary fruits and vegetables.

This is not true, because animals can produce vitamin C within their bodies, and in fact, human flesh contains it. First, if humans do not eat carbohydrates at all, enough vitamin C can be derived from lightly cooked meat and fat alone. Second, consuming less carbohydrates actually leads to the body needing less vitamin C, because carbohydrates actually compete with Vitamin C for access to the same metabolic pathways in the body; eating less carbohydrates means that the body needs less of Vitamin C. Lastly, there is a wide variety of many fresh, low- carbohydrate food sources such as dark leafy vegetables (e.g. broccoli, kale) as well as green and red peppers, that have high levels of vitamin C.

Myth #3: Ketogenic diets cause your body to go into ketosis, which is dangerous.

Most detractors cite this because they confuse ketosis with ketoacidosis. In a sensible ketogenic diet practiced by a healthy individual, ketosis is regulated by insulin, which controls the creation of ketone bodies and tightly regulates the flow of fatty acids into the blood. The insulin does not allow ketone bodies to reach toxic levels.

For people with metabolic issues, such as type 1 diabetics, where the body does not produce adequate amounts of insulin, it will not be able to regulate ketones in the same way as a healthy body can. Because there is no insulin to regulate the flow of ketones, ketones can accumulate in the blood, which turn the blood into an acidic and potentially deadly environment. This condition is called ketoacidosis. The signs of this condition generally appear within 24 hours of the accumulation of toxic ketone levels. It should be noted that ketoacidosis is a medical emergency, and if left untreated, can lead to loss of consciousness, and even death.

The levels of ketones associated with ketoacidosis are about three to five times higher than the levels associated with nutritional ketosis. So long as your ketone levels stay in a nutritional ketosis range, there is no risk for ketoacidosis. Still, some careful people will go ahead and measure the ketone levels in their blood. However, others will simply skip this step and eat the right food, assuming that they are going into the ketogenic state. In an overwhelming majority of dieters, this poses no health risk whatsoever.

There are blood and urine tests that can be done rather easily and cheaply if ketone levels are an issue while being on the ketogenic diet. Drugstores sell urine strips that indicate the level of ketones in urine. The strips measure the pH in urine and provides a good idea of your ketone levels.

For those who do not want to rely on urine testing, which is not nearly an accurate indicator over a longer period of time, blood meters may be used to measure ketone levels. The test requires simply pricking a finger with a lancet, and then placing the drop of blood on the included specialized testing strip, which will indicate the ketone levels.

Myth #4: Your kidneys will sustain damage from the high protein consumption.

This is a knee-jerk reaction to any low-carb diet, but the answer is that a Ketogenic diet is a high-fat diet, and not a high-protein one; and even if there is more protein in the diet than usual, there is plenty of scientific evidence that since it is a key nutrient in the prevention of osteoporosis. In fact, low protein shows that eating a little extra protein is perfectly safe, and will not harm the kidneys.

Myth #5: A high-fat diet will lead to osteoporosis, because it will cause the body to excrete calcium.

This once again stems from the misconception that the ketogenic diet is a high-protein diet. Anyway protein consumption is essential for good bone health, intake is often observed in patients with hip fractures. It has been observed that a deficiency in dietary protein causes a significant loss of bone mass and strength.

Myth #6: Eating Fat Makes You Fat

This seems like a no-brainer on the surface – after all, body fat should come from nowhere else, but fat. Actually, eating more fat causes us to eat less, as we have already found out. In the process of eating and metabolism, our body responds every time we think about food by having the pancreas secrete insulin. This in turn, tells your body to store fatty acids instead of using them for energy. Storing the fatty acids, instead of using them for energy, causes hunger; and when people get hungry, they eat.

In the famous "Chinese food" story, a typical lunch may consist of rice, noodles, and egg rolls – comprised of at least 70% carbohydrates, with a fortune cookie at the end, made up mostly of sugar and carbohydrates. This carbohydrate-packed meal passes through the digestive system quickly, causing significant spikes in blood sugar, and has virtually no fat. The body quickly breaks down this high- carbohydrate meal, and sends a sudden rush of glucose into the bloodstream. The body responds to this glucose rush by secreting more insulin, and helps carry the glucose from the blood into the cells. This causes the glucose levels in the bloodstream to drop, and hunger pangs set in again, causing the body to secrete more insulin, and the cycle starts over.

Myth #7: Cholesterol Causes Heart Disease

This erroneous theory comes from the even more erroneous concept that eating fat causes cholesterol build-up. First of all, cholesterol is absolutely essential for a human being's survival. This "lipoprotein" performs three important functions. First, it comprises bile acids that help you digest food; second, it allows the body to make vitamin D and other essential hormones such as estrogen and testosterone; and finally, it is one of the components of the outer coating of every one of your cells. Without this coating, the body would literally crumble.

Second, most of the cholesterol in the body does not come from what humans eat. Instead, about three-fourths is actually made in the body, with the other 25 percent coming from food. In addition, most of the cholesterol that is eaten passes right through the digestive tract and never even enters the bloodstream. This is the reason that the amount of cholesterol in the blood is tightly controlled by the body. When dietary cholesterol is eaten, the body shuts down its own production of cholesterol to compensate for this infusion.

Still, one in four people are hypersensitive to dietary cholesterol, although the increased cholesterol levels do not increase their risk of heart disease. A separate study published in the Journal of the American Medical Association reported findings that neither LDL nor HDL levels were important risk factors for death from coronary artery disease or heart attack. Even if someone were to go on a totally cholesterol-free diet, the body would simply compensate by increasing its cholesterol production by the liver to keep your blood levels steady. That's because, once again, your body needs cholesterol to survive.

Chapter Six
Warnings and Precautions

Like any other diet plan, there are things to watch out for when going on a Ketogenic diet. Some of the following precautions have serious consequences on overall body health.

Physiological adjustments

The first week on the ketogenic diet can be a very rough period. In this stage, the body is entering a state where it is burning ketones for energy, instead of glucose. This state can cause dizziness and lightheadedness and a general feeling of weakness. It can make you feel downright miserable. In many cases, these conditions persist until the second week, or even for a longer period, even if the body will eventually adjust to the ketogenic state. Obviously, medical attention should be sought if similar conditions worsen, or continue for much longer than two weeks.

There are other feelings of discomfort that may appear as a result of the body getting used to ketosis. This includes a metallic taste, or dryness, in the mouth, increased frequency in urinating, difficulty sleeping, increased thirst, and cold hands or feet.

Protein deficiency

There are concerns regarding what happens to amino acid production if someone on a ketogenic diet consumes dietary fat to the exclusion of dietary protein and carbohydrates. If someone's glucose requirements are high, such as someone who is very physically active, but glucose availability is low, the body will break down its protein from its storage in order to produce glucose via a process called gluconeogenesis. This is especially true in the initial days of fasting or starting a high fat diet. This has led some detractors to believe that a high-fat, ketogenic diet will lead to muscle loss and atrophy. However, someone on the Ketogenic diet can take in adequate protein, as they see fit, during the initial stages of the diet, to prevent muscle loss.

Overeating

While being it a state of ketosis means that excess fat is constantly being burned because of the absence of glucose, it is important note here that eating way too much of any food, including fat, will lead to weight gain. Constantly exceeding caloric needs will lead to weight gains, whether the overeating is done with carbohydrates, protein, or fat, although as we have seen, fat is not the major culprit when it comes to weight gain.

Alcohol

Alcohol is not good for the Ketogenic diet, and consumption of alcohol will almost completely impair the body's use of fat for fuel. Most alcohol products, especially beer, contain significant amounts of carbohydrates, which as we have seen, affects how fat is used as fuel by the body. Alcohol should be avoided at all times to ensure that the health benefits of the Ketogenic diet are maintained.

Patience

Some people lose a significant number of pounds during the first few weeks on the ketogenic diet. This causes many people to have unrealistic expectations while on this diet. As in any diet that leads to significant weight loss, weight drops are not uniform or even. Many find that they hit a disappointing "plateau," where it seems like they cannot shed any more pounds. It may be difficult to stay on the diet if the plateau extends for more than a few days, so some patience is called for. Some may find that while they continue to lose weight, it is not at the pace that was achieved at the beginning of the diet, and this may make it difficult for some to want to continue. Adjustments in the intake of other nutrients, a decrease in water intake, or increased physical activity, are some of the ways to get out of the plateau.

Keto "Flu"

Also called "low-carbohydrate flu", keto flu is a condition that affects people within the first few days of starting a ketogenic diet. The ketogenic diet actually does not cause the flu in the viral sense, but its symptoms closely resemble that of the flu. This "flu" is caused by altered hormonal states and hormonal imbalances caused by carbohydrate withdrawal. Sufferers from keto flu report basic flu-like symptoms that include headache, decreased appetite, nausea, upset stomach and abdominal cramps, diarrhea, dehydration (because of loss of water weight,) and lack of mental clarity and focus, or what is commonly called, "brain fog." The duration of symptoms varies, but will typically last anywhere from a couple of days to a week.

Bad Breath

Because the body creates acetone as a waste product during ketosis, it may result in bad breath as some of this acetone is released in your breath, emitting some kind of ammonia-like or fruity scent. This is also somewhat caused by the water loss, so the bad breath can somewhat be treated by drinking more water. Chewing fresh mint leaves or taking sugar-free breath fresheners can also help.

Changes in appetite

Many people who are used to eating a low-fat diet already find that eating the amount of fat required on this diet is difficult. Fat makes the body feel full, and some may find it difficult to eat enough calories to keep the body from starving, and from staying in a state of ketosis. The body is also being provided with plenty of fat and protein, which are both much more satiating than carbohydrates. In this stage, it is important that you eat even if you feel like you aren't hungry, and make sure that your body is getting enough calories and nutrients, especially in the transition period in the early part of the diet.

The ketogenic diet also requires a careful balancing of protein, carbohydrates, and fat to ensure that the body continues to burn ketones. If a person eats too much protein or carbohydrates, the body will break its ketone state, and come out of ketosis. When this happens, it will take up to another two weeks before the body can return to the correct state.

Carbohydrate addiction is a genuine problem. Some research shows that carbohydrates activate certain stimuli in the brain that can be dependence-forming and cause addiction. Carbohydrate addicts have uncontrollable cravings for carbohydrates, and when they do eat them, they tend to binge. In a carbohydrate addict, the removal of carbohydrates can cause withdrawal symptoms, such as dizziness and irritability, and intense cravings.

As your body adapts to a ketogenic diet, you may have a decreased appetite. The nausea associated with "keto flu" can also decrease your appetite.

Chapter Seven
Starting the Diet

Before even starting on the Ketogenic diet, remember that in the beginning, the diet can be difficult to maintain, even with amazing results. The first week or two on the diet can be rough, but doing the diet properly is insurance that weight loss and better health is guaranteed.

The signs that a body is in ketosis may start appearing even after only one week of following a true ketogenic diet. This is called, the "induction", or initial phase, in the famous Atkins diet, and during this period, fat and weight loss start to become evident. It can take longer for some people, even as much as three months, for the first effects to be felt. The amount of time it takes to start seeing signs that the body is burning fat for fuel largely depends on the individual. When signs do start to show, they are pretty similar across the board, and the weight loss is usually significant in the early stages.

Keep others involved

This diet can be very difficult for people who want to eat with other people. If people are unable to convince others to join them in the ketogenic diet, they often find that more than one meal must be prepared to keep just one person on the ketogenic diet. Hopefully, the commitment, determination, and success, will make others realize that the effort is worth their while, and they may even eventually try the diet. In fact, this diet can provide a great way to inform and educate others about the basics of food, nutrition, and the importance of eating a healthy diet.

Purchase a carbohydrate "guide"

A good carbohydrate guide is the first and probably, most helpful tool to use with the ketogenic diet, especially for those who are just starting out. Many books not only provide a list of foods and their carbohydrate count, but also show a certain food item's calorie, protein, and fat content. The more helpful books categorize foods according to type, such as meats, poultry, and seafood, among others.

Starting the diet - Which Ketogenic diet to start with

While the beneficial effects of the ketogenic diet can be enjoyed by practically 100% of the population, the diet can be applied in degrees, depending on how much, and how, carbohydrates are removed from an individual's diet. Determining the ideal type or level is done by evaluating the person's weight loss goals, lifestyle, and current physical condition. The only constant is that food eaten over the course of a day must be "balanced" from a ketogenic standpoint, so that they are high in fat, have adequate protein, and are extremely low in carbohydrates. There are at least four "types" or levels of the ketogenic diet that people can go on.

1) The standard ketogenic diet

This diet is a good choice for the vast majority of people. The main emphasis on this diet is to eat only between 30 and 50 grams of carbohydrates each day. If the person is more active, more carbohydrates, around up to 100 grams, can be consumed. For protein, the recommended quantity is between 115 grams and 175 grams per day. The rest of the diet should be concentrated on fat. For a 2,000 calorie daily diet, approximately 60% or 1,200 calories should come from fat, 25%, or 500 calories from protein, and 15%, or 300 calories, from carbohydrates.

2) The "targeted" ketogenic diet for overweight people

A second group that can benefit from the ketogenic diet are those individuals who are overweight, as the foods that are consumed on this diet are usually very low calorie. This type of ketogenic diet is also called "targeted ketogenic diet."

In this diet, a person needs to consume easily digestible carbohydrates with a high glycemic index within 60 minutes of exercising. Most people eating this diet are encouraged to eat a maximum of 25 grams of carbohydrates each day. Right after exercising, 30 grams of protein will be eaten. The protein intake is seen as particularly important because it helps to repair muscles that are injured during exercise.

People who have Type 2 Diabetes, as explained in Chapter 3, would also often find their condition improve because the diet avoids almost all kinds and types of sugar. However, diabetics who are insulin dependent should not start the ketogenic diet without consulting their doctors because going on this diet without carefully controlling the body's insulin levels can result in diabetic ketoacidosis (discussed in Chapter 5) that has been known to be fatal. Research also suggests that those individuals who have a higher cardiovascular risk factor because of arterial plaque, may benefit from type of ketogenic diet. Additional research needs to be done, but early findings suggest that people with brain cancer can benefit from this diet. Finally, many athletes find that their performance improves slightly after they have been on the diet for 12 weeks.

3) Cyclic diet for weightlifters and body builders

The third type of ketogenic diet is called, the "cyclic" ketogenic diet. This diet requires that people alternate between eating a low carbohydrate diet and a high carbohydrate diet. On the low carb days, it is recommended that people alternate eating 50 carbohydrates on "low carb" days, and between 450 and 600 grams of carbohydrates on high carb days. This form of the ketogenic diet is very popular with weightlifters and body builders because it maximizes fat loss and encourages the body to build lean mass. This diet must be carefully controlled by a dietician and should never be used just to have high carb meals several times a week.

4) Ketogenic diet for cancer patients

A fourth type of ketogenic diet is designed to help certain cancer patients. At the National Institutes of Health, researchers found that people who have certain types of cancer, particularly pancreatic cancer, can use the ketogenic diet to starve cancer cells in the body, by almost totally removing glucose from the diet. They discovered that by starving the cells of the glycogen, the cancerous cells apparently die. The diet is started with a three- to five-day water-only fast. After this fast, less than 20 grams of carbohydrates are eaten daily. Once again, this diet should only be done under a doctor's care, especially because of the extreme water diet at the beginning of the diet.

Regardless of which approach is used, the ketogenic diet can produce amazing results, if correctly applied. The great news for many dieters is that because of its high fat content, people seldom feel hungry.

Exercising

It is not recommended to start an exercise program while beginning the ketogenic diet. Note that all these diets rely on the same basic concept of getting carbohydrates down and stopping insulin production, which puts your body into fat-release-fat-burn mode. Exercising while energy sources in the body are being reconfigured is not a good idea, because the body will not yet have the energy required for it.

Remember that once you have reached ketosis, the desirable macro-nutrient ratio is around 65% fat, 20% protein, and 15% carbohydrates, for maintenance purposes.

Chapter Eight
What to Eat and What to Avoid

Shopping for the right foods correctly is the first, and most important step short of putting the right food in the mouth. For today's food shopper, this task is easier because fortunately, most food manufacturers are sensitive to the needs and requirements of people who go on special diets such as the ketogenic diet. Most food manufacturers and suppliers, in labeling their foods, have endeavored to be more accurate and responsive to people who need proper information to maintain strict diet regimens.

Regardless of whether foods are "allowed," the serious dieter will still have to make sure that they are staying well within the required macronutrient ratios (65% fat, 20% protein, and 15% carbohydrates). If measuring ratios are not possible during a given meal, the overriding principle is that the majority of the calories eaten daily should come from fat, and a very small percentage should be from carbohydrates.

Quality

The "quality" of your food matters, especially when it comes to fat and protein sources. Going back to the prehistoric template, our ancestors got healthy on unprocessed and unrefined food alone. It would be healthy and beneficial if a diet plan replicates that prehistoric food profile.

A ketogenic dieter should also try to purchase food that have the following descriptions on the labels: organic, grass-fed, free-range, and/or pasture-raised. Food with labels that say, "farm-raised" should be avoided as much as possible, because in all probability, whatever has been "raised" in those "farms" have been sprinkled with a healthy dose of chemicals and preservatives to improve yield and increase the animals' sizes.

Meats, poultry, and seafood

These are the staples of the ketogenic diet, not grains and rice. They are the most abundant, and in fact, flavorful components of the diet, and contains naturally-occurring fat. There are many foods in this category that most people can eat all they want daily. Foods included on this food group include all types of beef, chicken, turkey, ducks, fish, lamb, pork, shrimp, crab, and lobster. Of course, "exotic" varieties such as ostrich, deer, and buffalo, are also allowed, if available. While bacon and sausage are excellent sources of protein and fat, care should be taken in eating processed meats, especially hotdogs and sausages. Many brands contain significant amounts of carbohydrate fillers.

Remember that when eating meat, make sure to stay within your recommended protein grams for the day, since your body converts excess protein into glucose via glucogenesis, which can kick you out of the ketosis state.

Eggs

These should come from your local farmer or from pasture-raised, or free-range hens whenever possible. Omega-3 enriched eggs are especially recommended.

Vegetables and Fruits

In general, the greener and leafier the vegetable, the better, because this indicates that the food has a lower carbohydrate content. While most dieters on the ketogenic diet will want to get an extensive carbohydrate chart anyway, there is actually a relatively simple way to tell if you find yourself standing in the middle of the vegetable aisle without your list.

If the vegetable is a leaf, it contains almost no carbohydrates, and therefore, allowable. Most types of greens are encouraged, including spinach, lettuce, spinach, and mustard greens. If the vegetable grows as a stem or flower, it is also usually very low in carbohydrates. For example, radishes and mushrooms all have less than one gram of carbohydrates. Dieters can also eat all the celery and broccoli they want. If the vegetables contain seeds, then it is usually moderate in carbohydrates. If the vegetable grows as a root, like potatoes or yams, then it should probably be avoided because of its high starch content.

Most fruits are off limits on the ketogenic diet, especially citrus fruits, as well as most fruits that are easily convertible to juices, such as pineapple and mangoes. Even though the sugars in fruit are natural sugars, they still raise your blood glucose levels significantly and can kick you out of ketosis.

When you do eat fruit, choose fruits that are high in fiber and lower in carbohydrates, such as berries, which were extensively eaten by our prehistoric ancestors. For example, one-fourth cup of strawberries contains only about 1.5 grams of carbohydrates. Always remember that portion control is a necessity with carbohydrates, whether or not they are allowed. Avocados are one of the best fruits for the diet, with just one-half carb gram for an entire fruit.

Dairy

Full-fat dairy products can be a staple on the ketogenic diet. Butter, heavy cream, sour cream, cream cheese, hard cheese, and cottage cheese are very good in meeting fat intake needs. Grass-fed butter and organic creams, cheese, if at all possible, are highly recommended. Only whole fat milk should be ingested, if milk is desired. With the wide varieties of dairy products available, it is very important to read the food labels to ensure that there are no "hidden" carbohydrates. There is, for example, a big difference in carbohydrate content between cheese, and what is sold as, "cheese food," which contains just a small amount of cheese, but is full of carbohydrate fillers.

Avoid low-fat dairy products and flavored dairy products, such as fruity yogurt. Flavored yogurt is full of sugar; serving for serving, and some versions actually contain as much sugar and carbohydrates as sugared soda!

Beverages and alcohol

Dieters can also consume a variety of beverages on this diet in moderation, as long as they contain no sugar. Check the labels carefully on so-called diet sodas to make sure that they do not contain any sugars. Unlimited drinks will include tea, coffee, and heavy cream, minus any refined sugars or sweeteners. As with most diet plans , water is still the best bet as a beverage alternative - it is a good idea to drink at least half of your body weight in ounces. Plain water can be infused with fresh herbs, such as mint or basil, to provide a little variety. Sodas, flavored waters, sweetened teas, sweetened lemonade, and fruit juices should be avoided.

High-fructose corn-syrup, is that deadly stealth sweetener found in most soft drinks, and juices. If the "high" in high-fructose is not enough to scare someone away, consider that it also functions like a preservative, meaning that not only does it lack B vitamins and other important nutrients, it is chock-full of chemicals that have no business being in the human body.

Other fats and Oils

Allowable oils include as olive oil, and oils and butters derived from nuts. Try to avoid highly processed polyunsaturated fats, such as canola oil, vegetable oil, and soybean oil. Homemade mayonnaise is also an easy way to add a dose of fat to every meal.

Special fats: Medium-Chain-Triglycerides (MCT Oil)

There is even better news for ketogenic dieters: eating certain kinds of fat may leverage the already powerful effects of ketosis. Eating certain foods may increase the level of a "medium-chain" (referring to their chemical structure) fat that can deliver impressive metabolic and hormonal benefits. These are called Medium-Chain-Triglycerides, or MCT Oil, that in clinical trials, have been identified for possible applications to treat high-blood pressure and diabetes.

Many ketogenic advocates go as far as calling MCTs the ultimate ketogenic fat, because incorporating them to your diet not only helps in diabetes and hypertension, but is also said to create ketones to a degree that a ketogenic dieter can actually increase carbohydrate intake, while still remaining in ketosis.

Foods with higher levels of MCT are: coconut oil, oil from palm kernels, butter, cheese, yogurt, and whole milk.

The No-no's

Grains and Sugars

Avoid grains and sugars in all of their forms, while on the ketogenic diet. Grains include wheat, barley, rice, rye, sorghum, and anything made from these products. This means that the ketogenic diet will have no breads, no pasta, no crackers, and no rice. Sugar, and anything that contains sugar, is also not allowed on a ketogenic diet. This includes white sugar, brown sugar, honey, maple syrup, corn syrup, and brown rice syrup. There are many names for sugar on ingredient lists; it's extremely beneficial to become familiar with these names to know when a product contains sugar in any form. Be careful of artificial sweeteners like Splenda that could actually be made out of sucralose, which contains carbohydrates.

Packaged food and "T.V. dinners"

Boxed and frozen packaged dinners contain significant amounts of sugars, preservatives and chemicals, and should be avoided. These include dinners with big portions of meat products. Of course, breakfast pastries, hotcakes, waffles and toaster pastries are prohibited on the diet.

Candies, cakes, and desserts

Some varieties of these treats have enough carbohydrates in one serving to account for one week's worth of carbohydrate allocation. These should be avoided like the plague, although a few sugar-free items can be eaten. For desserts, "sugar-free" does not mean it is carbohydrate-free.

Conclusion to Book 1

Thank you again for reading this book!

I hope this book was able to help you understand and hopefully, get started with the ketogenic diet.

Success on the ketogenic diet will take some commitment. You also need to be careful when making food choices. However, so long as a dieter stays within the required macronutrient ratios, some trial and error is tolerable.

Once a dieter gets into the routine, and food selection and intake becomes automatic, a state of optimal ketosis will be achieved, and the body will adjust accordingly.

Just remember to seek a medical professional if any uncomfortable symptom arises, or if a medical condition exists that you are not sure about. A qualified nutritionist can also be helpful for any "troubleshooting" issues, if and when results are not arriving as expected. Enjoy your voyage to a healthy lifestyle!

Finally, if you enjoyed this book, then I'd like to ask you for a favor, would you be kind enough to leave a review for this book on Amazon? It'd be greatly appreciated!

You can do so by typing this link into your browser:

→ bit.ly/KetoReview ←

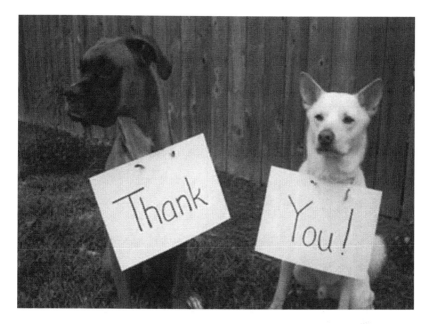

Thank you and good luck!

Free Bonus!

As you know, reading this book alone will not guarantee you any results. As with any goal, you must take action and stay motivated in the long term. For this reason, I've created an exclusive club for us to help each other on our ketogenic journeys, keep each other motivated and share each other's success. Together we can achieve the results we want!

I'm also giving away a FREE 30 Day Diet Plan Book with 90 of the tastiest Ketogenic Recipes for members only!

You can join The Ketogenic Dieters' Club for FREE by typing this link into your browser:

→ bit.ly/KetoClub ←

See you on the inside! – Oliver

In the meantime, continue reading for The Ketogenic Cookbook!

The Ketogenic Cookbook

The Top 50 Ketogenic Recipes

Oliver Ryan

SCHOFIELD PUBLISHING HOUSE

TABLE OF CONTENTS

Breakfast Recipes

TABLE OF CONTENTS

Lunch Recipes

TABLE OF CONTENTS

Dinner Recipes

TABLE OF CONTENTS

Dessert Recipes

TABLE OF CONTENTS

Snack Recipes

Ketogenic Breakfast Recipes

Quick Egg Scramble with Dry Salami

Time: 10 minutes   Servings: 1

Ingredients

- 2 eggs
- 50g dry salami
- 1 tsp rosemary
- 150g ricotta cheese

- 1 tbsp olive oil
- Salt
- Pepper

Directions

1. Cut salami in small pieces adds olive oil in pan and fry salami pieces.

2. Break the egg into another pan and whisk it.

3. Then add rosemary, salt and pepper as per your taste.

4. Then include ricotta cheese into egg mixture and mix well without any lumps.

5. Add egg and ricotta mixture into pan and cook until 5 minutes.

6. After 5 minutes add fry salami pieces into pan and serve hot.

Nutritional Value per Serving

Protein: 28g   Fat: 45g   Carbs: 5g   Kcal: 598

Crisp and Crunchy Crust Cheddar

Time: 12 minutes   Servings: 1

Ingredients

- 2 slice cheddar cheese
- 1 egg
- 1 tsp almond powder
- 1 tbsp olive oil

- 1 tsp hemp seed
- 1 tsp flax seed ground
- Salt and pepper as per taste

Directions

1. Add tablespoon olive oil into pan and turn on medium heat.

2. Break the egg and add salt and pepper into them and whisk about 1 minute.

3. Add ground flax seed into almond flour and hemp seed.

4. Dip the cheddar cheese slice into egg mixture, then coat with the dry mixture.

5. Then fry 4 minute both the side and serve hot.

Nutritional Value per Serving

Protein:	Fat:	Carbs:	Kcal:	Fiber:
35g	48g	5g	588	2g

Low-Carb Cheese Pancakes

Time: 15 minutes   Servings: 4

Ingredients

- 2 eggs
- 55g cream cheese

- 1 tsp castor sugar
- ½ tsp cinnamon

Directions

1. Put in all ingredients into blender and blend until it forms smooth mixture.

2. After that take pan and grease them with butter and add ¼ of batter into hot pan.

3. Then cook 2 minutes until its golden, after 2 minutes flip and cook 1 minute other side.

4. Serve hot with berries and your choice sugar free syrup.

4

Nutritional Value per Serving

Protein: 17g   Fat: 29g   Carbs: 2.5g   Kcal: 344

Healthy Low-Carb Waffles

Time: 15 minutes   Servings: 1

Ingredients

- 2 egg whites
- 2 tbsp milk
- 2 tbsp coconut flour

- ½ tsp baking powder
- 1 tbsp castor sugar

Directions

1. Take a bowl and whisk egg whites until it form stiff.

2. Once it will stiff then add coconut flour, milk, castor sugar and baking powder.

3. Now softly fold all mixture together.

4. Now take waffle mixture and place into the waffle maker to make waffle.

5. Cook until it forms golden.

6. Serve waffles with low-carb ice-cream and some berries.

Nutritional Value per Serving

Protein: 25g   Fat: 3.5g   Carbs: 2g   Kcal: 121

Keto Omelet with Fried Avocado

Time: 12 minutes   Servings: 4

Ingredients

- 4 eggs
- 55g cheese
- 1 tsp herbs
- 1 avocado

- 10 olives
- 2 tbsp oil
- 2 tbsp butter
- ½ tsp salt

Directions

1. Break the egg in large bowl and whisk with oil, herbs, olive and salt until it forms frothy.

2. Peel the avocado and make thick slices.

3. Add butter in pan with high flame then add avocado slices in the pan and fry until it forms golden both side.

4. Then remove avocado slices in the plate and set aside.

5. Now pour the egg mixture in the pan and cook 3 minute until the bottom forms golden brown.

6. Now serve omelet in large plate with fried avocado.

Nutritional Value per Serving

Protein: 9g   Fat: 30g   Carbs: 2g   Kcal: 313

Gluten Free Pumpkin Pancake

Time: 40 minutes   Servings: 6

Ingredients

- 3 eggs
- 25 gm egg white protein
- 55g hazelnut flour
- 55g ground flax seed
- 1 tsp baking powder

- 1 tsp vanilla
- 1 cup coconut cream
- ½ cup pumpkin puree
- 4 drop sweetener
- Oil

Directions

1. Add all wet ingredients in bowl and whisk until frothy.

2. Take another bowl and add the flour, baking powder and sweetener.

3. Add dry mixture slowly to wet mixture as you keep whisking. Whisk slowly until batter is ready it should be thick but pourable.

4. If it looks dry then add ¼ cup of water.

5. After that take pan and grease them with oil and pour scoop of batter into hot pan.

6. Cover a pan with lid and cook the pancakes about 3 minutes both the side.

7. Serve immediately with cream of your choice.

Nutritional Value per Serving

Protein: 21g   Fat: 35g   Carbs: 4g   Kcal: 413   Fiber: 7g

Low-Carb Cheddar Cheese Soufflés

Time: 35 minutes   Servings: 7

Ingredients

- 6 eggs separated
- ½ cup almond flour
- ¼ tsp chili pepper
- 1 tsp ground mustard
- 2 cup shredded cheddar cheese

- ¾ cup cream
- ½ tsp ground flax seed
- ¼ cup chopped chives
- ½ tsp black pepper
- Salt

Directions

1. Preheat the oven 360F and grease the soufflé mold and set aside on cookie sheet.

2. Take a large bowl add in almond flour, salt, mustard, ground flex seed, chili pepper and mix it well.

3. Then add cream, cheese, chives, egg yolks and whisk slowly until all ingredients incorporated.

4. Now take another bowl and beat egg white until it forms stiff after that add slowly egg white stiff mixture into the almond and cheese mixture and fold with carefully until it combine.

5. Pour the mixture into the grease soufflé mold and put the cookie sheet into the preheated oven.

6. Bake the soufflé about 25 minute or golden brown.

7. Serve hot.

Nutritional Value per Serving
Protein: 15g   Fat: 25g   Carbs: 2g   Kcal: 213   Fiber: 2g

Yummy Mozzarella Tacos

Time: 35 minutes   Servings: 3

Ingredients

- 6 eggs

- 2 tbsp butter

- 3 bacon strip

- ½ avocado

- 1 cup shredded mozzarella cheese

- 28g shredded cheddar cheese

- Salt

- Pepper

Directions

1. Cook bacon in the oven about 20 minutes at 350F.

2. Now heat 1/3 cup of mozzarella in the pan for taco shells and cook about 3 minutes until it forms brown.

3. Now lift the cheese shells with the help of sandwich tongs and drape it over the spoon resting on a pot.

4. Then cook egg in butter with seasoning of salt and pepper.

5. Now add one spoon scrabbled egg, avocado and bacon in harden taco shell.

6. Sprinkle some cheddar cheese over the top also adds sauce and cilantro if you like.#

Nutritional Value per Serving
Protein: 26g   Fat: 36g   Carbs: 3g   Kcal: 440

Coconut and Blueberry Pudding

Time: 35 minutes   Servings: 2

Ingredients

- 5 egg yolks
- 2 tbsp butter
- ¼ cup coconut flour
- ¼ tsp baking powder
- 2 tbsp coconut oil
- 2 tbsp fat cream

- 1 lemon zest
- 2 tsp lemon juice
- ¼ cup blueberries
- 2 tbsp powder sugar
- 9 drops liquid sweetener

Directions

1. Preheat the oven 360F.

2. Take egg yolks in bowl and whisk until light in color then add powder sugar and liquid sweetener. Whisk again until combine well.

3. Now add fat cream, lemon zest, lemon juice, coconut oil and butter. Whisk again until combine well.

4. Divide batter in two molds and add 2 tbsp blueberries in each mold.

5. Put the mold into oven and bake about 20-25 minute, let it cool and enjoy.

Nutritional Value per Serving

Protein: 9g   Fat: 44g   Carbs: 4.5g   Kcal: 470

Keto Cheese and Spinach Egg Scramble

Time: 15 minutes   Servings: 1

Ingredients

- 4 eggs
- ½ cup cheddar cheese
- 4 cup spinach
- 1 tbsp fat cream

- 1 tbsp olive oil
- Salt
- Pepper

Directions

1. Break 4 eggs in large bowl and add 1 tbsp fat cream and salt and pepper as per taste.

2. Take a large pan and heat high with 1 tbsp olive oil. When oil reach smoke point then add spinach and sprinkle some seasoning salt, pepper.

3. Once spinach has wilted then reduce heat medium and add eggs mixture.

4. Mix slowly once egg set then add cheddar cheese wait until cheese melted.

5. Serve hot immediately and enjoy.

Nutritional Value per Serving

Protein: 40g   Fat: 55g   Carbs: 5g   Kcal: 630   Fiber: 3g

Ketogenic Lunch Recipes

Healthy Low-Carb Stuffed Cucumber

Time: 10 minutes   Servings: 2

Ingredients

- 1 peeled cucumber
- 1 tsp olive oil
- 2 tbsp cream cheese
- 1 tsp vinegar

- 1 chopped tomato
- ½ mashed avocado
- 28g chopped hot chili pepper

Directions

1. Take a peeled cucumber and make two half pieces. Then remove center seed from cucumber and set aside.

2. Then take bowl and add olive oil, cream cheese, vinegar, chopped tomato, mashed avocado and chili pepper and blend all together until get smooth paste.

3. Add paste in piping bag and pipe paste in cucumber.

4. Now make ½ inches slice of cucumber and serve.

Nutritional Value per Serving

Protein: 8g   Fat: 26g   Carbs: 3g   Kcal: 170   Fiber: 3g

Cream Cheese Chicken Soup

Time: 10 minutes   Servings: 1

Ingredients

- 113g cream cheese
- 2 cup shredded chicken, cooked
- 1/3 cup hot sauce
- 3 tbsp butter

- 4 cup chicken broth
- ¼ cup celery
- Salt
- Pepper

Directions

1. Add cream cheese, butter, chicken stock and hot sauce in blender and blend until get smooth puree.

2. Now add this puree in saucepan and cook until it hot does not boil the puree.

3. Then take serving bowl add hot puree in it now add shredded chicken and celery.

4. Sprinkle some seasoning salt and pepper as per your taste and enjoy.

Nutritional Value per Serving

Protein: 30g   Fat: 28g   Carbs: 5g   Kcal: 403

Keto Low-Carb Fried Chicken

Time: 135 minutes   Servings: 7

Ingredients

- 6lbs chicken leg
- 1 cup coconut flour
- 1 tsp salt
- 1 tsp garlic powder
- 1 tsp pepper
- 1 tsp paprika
- Oil for fry

Directions

1. Add chicken in large bowl for marinade then add garlic powder, salt, paprika and pepper mix all them about 5 minute after that cover bowl and refrigerate for 2 hours.

2. After 2 hours take marinade chicken bowl and add coconut flour and toss well until chicken coat.

3. Now take oil in deep pan when oil is ready to fry then add chicken in batches and fry about 8 minutes each side until it golden brown.

4. Serve Hot and enjoy.

Nutritional Value per Serving

Protein: 35g   Fat: 31g   Carbs: 2g   Kcal: 420

Cheese and Bacon Meatballs

Time: 120 minutes   Servings: 5

Ingredients

- 4 bacon slice
- 1/3 cup pork rinds crushed
- 1 ½ lb ground beef
- 1 cup mozzarella cheese
- 2 eggs

- 2 tsp garlic paste
- 1 tsp pepper
- ½ tsp onion powder
- ½ tsp salt

Directions

1. Preheat the oven at 360F temperature.

2. Chop bacon in small pieces then add ground beef, cheese, spices, pork rind and egg in the bacon. Then mix all ingredients about 5 minute.

3. Now make round meatballs and place into baking tray.

4. Bake the meatball in oven about 45 minutes or until bacon is cooked.

5. Serve hot meatball with your choice sauce and enjoy.

Nutritional Value per Serving

Protein: 11g   Fat: 10g   Carbs: 1g   Kcal: 130

Low-Carb Chicken Patties

Time: 30 minutes   Servings: 5

Ingredients

- 1 egg
- 1 chicken breast
- 2 bell peppers
- ¼ cup tomato pesto

- ¼ cup cheese
- 3 tbsp coconut flour
- 4 bacon slice

Directions

1. Add oil in pan and fry bacon both the side until it crisp.

2. Then add bacon and chop chicken in blender and blend until smooth. Now add this mixture in bowl.

3. Then add chopped bell pepper.

4. Now add tomato pesto, cheese, egg and coconut flour and mix together.

5. After that make patties with hand and fry in pan both side until it golden brown.

6. Serve hot with the sauce and enjoy.

Nutritional Value per Serving

Protein: 10g   Fat: 12g   Carbs: 1.6g   Kcal: 160

Bacon, Chicken and Spinach Salad

Time: 12 minutes   Servings: 1

Ingredients

- 1 egg boil
- 2 bacon strip
- 1 cup spinach
- 56g chicken breast

- ½ tomatoes
- ½ tsp vinegar
- ¼ avocado
- 1 tbsp olive oil

Directions

1. Take a cook chicken and bacon then chop bacon and chicken in small pieces.

2. Now chop avocado, spinach and tomato in small pieces.

3. Take a bowl and add chop chicken and bacon also add chop avocado, spinach and tomato.

4. Add olive oil and vinegar in bowl.

5. Mix well and enjoy.

Nutritional Value per Serving

Protein: 40g   Fat: 47g   Carbs: 3g   Kcal: 590

Simple Tuna Salad

Time: 15 minutes   Servings: 4

Ingredients

- 225g tuna
- 108g olive oil
- 1 cup feta cheese crumbled
- ½ cups roasted red pepper chopped

- ¼ cup green olives
- ¼ cup chopped parsley
- 1 tbsp lemon juice
- Black pepper
- Salt

Directions

1. Crumble tuna in the mixing bowl.

2. Add crumble cheese, roasted red pepper, olive oil, chopped parsley, olives and lemon juice. Mix very well to combine.

3. Season with black pepper and salt.

4. Serve immediately and enjoy.

Nutritional Value per Serving

Protein: 19g   Fat: 37g   Carbs: 2.5g   Kcal: 410

Spinach and Bell Pepper Quiche

Time: 20 minutes   Servings: 6

Ingredients

- 283g frozen chopped spinach
- ¾ cup shredded cheese
- ¾ cup liquid egg substitute
- ¼ cup chopped green bell pepper
- ¼ cup chopped onions

Directions

1. Microwave the spinach for 2 minutes on high.

2. Then line 12 cup muffin pan with foil baking cups. Grease the cup with cooking spray.

3. Add the egg substitute, peppers, cheese, spinach and onions in bowl.

4. Mix well and divide among the muffin cup.

5. Bake at 360F for 20 minutes, and enjoy.

Nutritional Value per Serving

Protein: 10g   Fat: 12g   Carbs: 1.5g   Kcal: 77

Low-Carb Tuna Patties

Time: 25 minutes   Servings: 4

Ingredients

- 225g tuna
- 1 egg
- ¼ cup almond flour
- 2 tbsp mayonnaise

- 27g olive oil
- 55g butter
- Salt
- Pepper

Directions

1. Combine tuna, mayonnaise, egg, almond flour, olive oil, salt and pepper in a bowl. And combine well.

2. Take a non-stick pan and melt the butter over medium heat.

3. Now take quarter of tuna mixture and make round patties on hand and cook in pan both side about 4 minute each side or until it golden brown.

4. Serve hot with the sauce and enjoy.

Nutritional Value per Serving

Protein: 14g   Fat: 30g   Carbs: 1g   Kcal: 320

Yummy Ham Puffs

Time: 40 minutes   Servings: 6

Ingredients

- 4 eggs
- ¼ cup coconut flour
- ½ cup mayonnaise
- ¼ cup oil

- ¼ tsp baking powder
- ¼ tsp baking soda
- 198g ham sliced
- 1 cup shredded cheddar cheese

Directions

1. Grease nonstick doughnut shape pan.

2. Preheat the oven 370F.

3. Take a bowl and whisk eggs, oil and mayonnaise.

4. Now stir in the coconut flour, baking soda and baking powder to the wet mixture.

5. Then fold ham and cheese into batter mix well and break lumps. Now fill the about three quarter batter in the pan and bake about 30 minutes.

6. Serve hot and enjoy.

Nutritional Value per Serving

Protein: 17g   Fat: 36g   Carbs: 3g   Kcal: 400

Ketogenic Dinner Recipes

Spicy Chicken Cheese Casserole

Time: 60 minutes   Servings: 6

Ingredients

- 6 bacon slice
- 6 chicken thighs
- 3 jalapenos
- 340g cream cheese
- 113g shredded cheddar cheese

- ¼ cup mayonnaise
- 56g shredded mozzarella cheese
- ¼ cup red hot sauce
- Salt
- Pepper

Directions

1. Preheat the oven at 400F.

2. Take chicken thighs remove the bone and season with salt and pepper and bake in preheated oven about 40 minutes.

3. Now add small chopped bacon into pan and on medium heat when bacon is crisped then add jalapenos into the pan.

4. Once jalapenos are soft then add mayonnaise, cream cheese and red hot sauce and mix all together well.

5. Now remove chicken from oven and let it cool once chicken is cool remove the chicken skin.

6. Take one casserole dish and add chicken in dish now add cream cheese mixture and spread on top mozzarella cheese and cheddar cheese.

7. Then bake about 15 minutes and serve hot immediately.

Nutritional Value per Serving
Protein: 32g   Fat: 60g   Carbs: 2.5g   Kcal: 730

Low-Carb Beef Stew

Time: 130 minutes   Servings: 4

Ingredients

- 945g beef broth
- 450g stew meat
- 55g butter
- 450g sliced mushroom
- 80g sliced onion
- 1 tsp garlic paste
- 1 tbsp flex seed ground

- 1tsp dried thyme
- ¼ cup fresh chopped parsley
- 2 bay leaves
- 108g olive oil
- Salt
- Pepper

Directions

1. Add butter and olive oil in heavy pot over medium heat to high heat until butter completely melted. Now add meat and cook until its color browned.

2. Now add mushroom and onion in pot and sauté until mushroom is soft.

3. Then add broth, garlic, thyme, flex seed and bay leaves and mix well and cooked about 2 hours until meat are tender.

4. Then remove bay leaves and shred the chunk of meat before serving.

5. Add fresh parsley and serve.

Nutritional Value per Serving

Protein: 27g   Fat: 58g   Carbs: 5g   Kcal: 640

Keto Chicken Curry

Time: 35 minutes   Servings: 6

Ingredients

- 450g chicken breast sliced
- 1 tbsp curry powder
- ½ cup onion
- 6 tbsp coconut oil
- 2 tsp garlic paste
- 2 tsp chopped ginger root
- 400g coconut milk
- 56g roasted peanut
- ¼ cup chopped cilantro
- Salt

Directions

1. Heat coconut oil in pan on medium heat. Add onion and curry powder and sauté until onion are soft.

2. Add sliced chicken and sauté. Now add garlic and ginger and combine well.

3. Then pour coconut milk and water over the chicken add some roasted peanut and mix well.

4. Cook chicken curry about 10 minutes, curry should be thickened and chicken cooked.

5. Now add freshly chopped cilantro and stir well.

6. Serve hot chicken curry with plain rice and enjoy.

Nutritional Value per Serving

Protein: 20g   Fat: 34g   Carbs: 4.5g   Kcal: 395

Cheese Stuffed Green Peppers

Time: 35 minutes   Servings: 2

Ingredients

- 2 green peppers
- 42g parmesan cheese
- 56g cream cheese

- 1 onion
- 2 sausages
- 1 egg

Directions

1. Remove skin of sausage and crumble them in pan and cook.

2. Then cut the top of the pepper and remove all seed.

3. Now chop the top of pepper in small pieces also chop onion and cook chop onion and pepper.

4. Then mix cheese, onion, pepper, sausage and cream cheese and mix all together.

5. Add egg in the mixture and combine all together and cook 5 minutes.

6. Now stuffed the mixture in pepper and sprinkle some parmesan cheese over the top.

7. Bake the stuffed pepper about 15 minutes and serve hot.

Nutritional Value per Serving

Protein: 30g   Fat: 36g   Carbs: 5g   Fiber: 3   Kcal: 480

Quick Baked Aioli Fish

Time: 30 minutes   Servings: 1

Ingredients

- 172g mild white fish
- 7g parmesan cheese grated
- 2 tbsp aioli

Directions

1. Preheat the oven at 360F. And take a nonstick pan and grease the pan with oil then spread fillet thickly with aioli and sprinkle parmesan cheese over on top.

3. Now turn fillet other side and sprinkle remaining parmesan cheese. Then bake for 20 minutes.

4. Then serve hot with steam rice and enjoy.

Nutritional Value per Serving

Protein: 33g   Fat: 21g   Carbs: 1g   Kcal: 190

Spicy Shrimp in Butter

Time: 30 minutes   Servings: 4

Ingredients

- 650g shrimp
- 85g butter
- 2 tsp cayenne
- ¾ tsp dried thyme
- ¾ tsp salt

- ½ tsp ground rosemary
- 6 garlic clove, crushed
- ½ tsp oregano
- 180ml light beer

Directions

1. Take a heavy pan and add butter in it when butter is melted then add salt, cayenne, thyme, ground rosemary, oregano and crushed garlic and mix well.

2. Then add shrimp in the pan and sauté about 5 minutes.

3. Now pour the light beer in the pan, cover the pan and let the shrimp cook about 3 minutes then remove pan cover and cook another 3 minutes.

4. Now remove the shrimp in serving bowl.

5. Then turn on the high heat under the pan and boil the sauce until reduced by about half and pour it over the shrimp.

6. Serve hot immediately and enjoy.

Nutritional Value per Serving

Protein: 39g   Fat: 25g   Carbs: 4g   Fiber: 2g   Kcal: 210

Simple Roasted Chicken

Time: 130 minutes   Servings: 5

Ingredients

- 1.5kg chicken
- 120ml olive oil
- 60ml lemon juice

- ¼ tsp pepper
- ½ tsp salt

Directions

1. Take bowl and add chicken then add lemon juice, olive oil, pepper and salt and mix them together after that cover bowl and refrigerate for 1 hour.

2. Then preheat oven at 370F

3. Now take marinated chicken and place into baking tray.

4. Roast chicken in oven about 1 hour or until it turns brown.

5. Serve hot and enjoy.

Nutritional Value per Serving

Protein: 52g   Fat: 35g   Carbs: 1g   Kcal: 351

Cheese and Smoked Salmon Scramble

Time: 30 minutes   Servings: 3

Ingredients

- 4 eggs
- 115g goat cheese
- 120ml fat cream
- 4 spring onion

- 1 tsp dried dill weed
- 115g smoked salmon
- 2 tbsp butter

Directions

1. Whisk egg, cream and dill weed together

2. Slice the spring onion also chops goat cheese in small pieces and make crumbles of smoked salmon.

3. Now take a pan, melt the butter over medium heat when the butter is melted add spring onion and sauté them about 2 minutes.

4. Then add egg mixture and cook stirring frequently until the eggs are half set about 2 minute.

5. Finally add goat cheese and smoked salmon continue stirring until eggs are set, and serve.

Nutritional Value per Serving

Protein: 26g   Fat: 28g   Carbs: 3g   Kcal: 371

Keto Mustard Salmon Steaks

Time: 120 minutes   Servings: 2

Ingredients

- 2 salmon steaks
- 1 tsp mustard
- 1 tbsp lemon juice

- 2 tbsp butter
- 1 pinch salt
- 2 tbsp chopped parsley

Directions

1. Add butter, mustard, lemon juice and salt in slow cooker. Set heat low and cook about 35 minutes and stir together.

2. Now add salmon steak in slow cooker and recover the slow cooker and let it cook about 60 minutes.

3. Sprinkle some freshly chopped parsley and serve hot.

Nutritional Value per Serving

Protein: 45g   Fat: 27g   Carbs: 1g   Kcal: 410

Pork Chop with Balsamic Vinegar

Time: 80 minutes   Servings: 2

Ingredients

- 3 pork chops
- ¾ cup chicken broth
- 2 tbsp olive oil

- 3 tbsp balsamic vinegar
- ¼ tsp guar
- 3 crushed garlic cloves

Directions

1. Take a large pan and put on medium-high heat add oil and chop and cook the both side until well browned.

2. Now add Vinegar, chicken broth and garlic in pan and cover the pan, turn the heat low and let the chop simmer for 60 minutes.

3. Then remove the chops in serving plate.

4. Now put pan liquid in blender and add guar then blend about 5 minute and pour thickened sauce over the chop and serve.

Nutritional Value per Serving

Protein: 36g   Fat: 29g   Carbs: 2g   Kcal: 340

Ketogenic Dessert Recipes

Low-Carb Chocolate Fudge

Time: 30 minutes   Servings: 16

Ingredients

- 55g melted chocolate
- 450g cream cheese
- 12g sweetener
- ½ cup chopped walnut
- 1 tsp vanilla extract

Directions

1. Blend Cream cheese until smooth. Then beat chocolate, vanilla and sweetener.

2. Then add chopped walnut and stir well.

3. Now take a pan 20*20cm with foil and smooth the cream cheese mixture into the pan.

4. Then Chill well and cut square pieces and enjoy.

Nutritional Value per Serving

Protein: 5g   Fat: 16g   Carbs: 1g   Kcal: 124

Blackberry Cups

Time: 35 minutes   Servings: 5

Ingredients

- 100g frozen blackberries
- 240ml boiling water
- 2 tsp lemon juice
- 1 package sugar free raspberry gelatin

- ½ grated orange rind
- 240ml heavy cream
- ½ tsp vanilla extract

Directions

1. Add water, lemon juice, gelatin and orange rind in blender and blend about 1 minute to dissolve gelatin.

2. Then add blackberries and blend again until mix the berries.

3. Now put blender container in the refrigerator about 10 minutes.

4. After 10 minutes add ¾ cup heavy cream and blend about 2 minutes. Then pour cream mixture in 5 little dessert cup and chill.

5. Then whip remaining cream with vanilla and serve.

Nutritional Value per Serving

Protein: 8g   Fat: 18g   Carbs: 1.5g   Fiber: 1g   Kcal: 172

Simple Vanilla pudding

Time: 35 minutes   Servings: 2

Ingredients

- 4 egg yolks
- 3 tsp sweetener
- 2 cup heavy cream

- 2 tsp arrowroot flour
- 1 tsp vanilla extract
- Pinch of salt

Directions

1. Take a bowl and add egg yolks, sweetener, heavy cream, arrowroot flour, vanilla extract and pinch of salt then whisk until egg yolks are combine well.

2. Then pour mixture in heavy-bottom pot and place the pot on medium heat then stir constantly. Once mixture being steam reduce the heat to low.

3. Then continue the cooking about 10 minutes.

4. After 10 minutes pour the pudding mixture in small cups. Let it cool for about 15 minutes and serve warm.

Nutritional Value per Serving

Protein: 4g   Fat: 24g   Carbs: 2g   Kcal: 230

Keto Peanut Butter Cookies

Time: 20 minutes   Servings: 16

Ingredients

- 1 egg

- 3 tsp sweetener

- 2 tsp coconut flour

- 115g butter, room temperature

- 130g peanut butter, unsweetened

Directions

1. Preheat the oven at 350F.

2. Line baking tray with parchment paper.

3. Take a bowl and add egg, sweetener, coconut flour, peanut butter and butter and mix all ingredients by using electric hand mixer.

4. Now make 16 small cookie and place into baking tray.

5. Bake cookie about 13 minutes until edges should be golden brown and crispy.

6. Allow cookie to cool about 5 minutes.

Nutritional Value per Serving

Protein: 5g   Fat: 12g   Carbs: 1.12g   Kcal: 104

Chocolate Chip Brownies

Time: 35 minutes   Servings: 16

Ingredients

- 2 eggs
- 115g butter
- ½ tsp salt
- 1 tbsp instant coffee crystals
- 45g cocoa powder

- 30g almond meal
- 65g vanilla protein powder
- 25g sweetener
- 170g chocolate chips
- 60ml water

Directions

1. Preheat the oven at 350F. Then add protein powder, sweetener, cocoa, almond meal, salt and coffee crystal in bowl and combine well.

3. Then add butter in bowl and beat with the electric hand mixer until the butter combine with dry ingredients.

4. Now add egg one at a time and beat well with a whisk. Then beat in the water.

5. Finally add chocolate chip in batter and stir well. Then add batter in greased nonstick tray.

6. Bake for 20 minutes. Cool and cut into square pieces.

Nutritional Value per Serving

Protein: 4g   Fat: 14g   Carbs: 1.5g   Kcal: 130

Keto Sugarless Chocolate Sauce

Time: 15 minutes   Servings: 1

Ingredients

- 55g baking chocolate
- 100g maltitol
- 3 tbsp butter
- ¼ tsp vanilla
- 80ml water

Directions

1. Add chocolate and water in bowl and place bowl into in microwave on high about 2 minute or until chocolate is melted.

2. Then add maltitol and microwave on high another 3 minute.

3. Add butter and vanilla and stir once. Now it is ready to serve.

Nutritional Value per Serving

Protein: 4g   Fat: 35g   Carbs: 3g   Kcal: 470

Low-Carb Chocolate Walnut Cookies

Time: 15 minutes   Servings: 35

Ingredients

- 1 egg
- 1 tsp vanilla extract
- 120g soy powder
- ¼ tsp salt
- 1 ½ tsp baking powder
- 55g baking chocolate

- ½ cup chopped walnut
- 2 tbsp sweetener
- ½ cup castor sugar
- 55g cream cheese
- 115g butter

Directions

1. Preheat the oven at 370F.

2. Beat the cream cheese and butter until soft and combine together.

3. Then add castor sugar, sweetener, egg and vanilla extract and beat until well combined.

4. Now sift the soy powder, salt and baking powder.

5. Add sifted powder mixture into the butter mixture.

6. Finally add melted chocolate and walnut in mixture and mix well.

7. Now grease the baking tray with butter and make small cookies of dough and place into the tray.

8. Bake cookies 10 minutes until brown or edges should be crispy.

Nutritional Value per Serving
Protein: 5g   Fat: 14g   Carbs: 1g   Kcal: 65   Fiber: 1g

Easy Blueberry Cheesecake

Time: 30 minutes   Servings: 8

Ingredients

- 6 eggs
- 120g cream cheese
- 1 tsp vanilla
- 150g melted butter

- ½ tsp baking powder
- ½ cup frozen blueberries
- 3 tbsp sweetener

Directions

1. Add eggs, cream cheese, vanilla, butter, baking powder and sweetener in bowl and beat it well until get smooth mixture.

2. Grease 20inch baking tray with butter and pour batter in it.

3. Now add frozen blueberries in batter and slightly mix.

4. Bake at 330F for 30 minutes until cake cook from center.

5. Allow cool then cut into pieces and serve.

Nutritional Value per Serving

Protein: 5g   Fat: 20g   Carbs: 1.5g   Kcal: 210   Fiber: 0.5g

Keto Chocolate Ice Cream

Time: 35 minutes   Servings: 8

Ingredients

- 3 eggs
- 1 cup cocoa powder
- 1 cup almond milk

- 1 cup granulated sugar substitute
- 1 ½ cup whipping cream
- Salt

Directions

1. Add eggs, Sugar substitute, almond milk and cocoa powder in blender and blend until smooth.

2. Add Mixture in bowl and microwave on high for about 1 minute.

3. Now stir mixture and microwave about 30 second. Stir well until remove lumps.

4. Now whisk in whipping cream and salt.

5. Then chill in refrigerator overnight.

6. Serve chilled ice cream with chocolate sauce or chocolate chips.

Nutritional Value per Serving

Protein: 6g   Fat: 23g   Carbs: 2g   Kcal: 230

Low-Carb Coffee Mousse

Time: 15 minutes   Servings: 10

Ingredients

- ½ cup hot brewed coffee
- 2 cup ricotta cheese
- 1 tsp instant espresso
- 2 ½ tsp dry gelatins
- 1 tsp vanilla liquid sweetener
- 1 cup whipping cream
- 1 tsp vanilla extract
- Salt

Directions

1. Add gelatin in hot coffee and stir well set aside until cool.

2. Add cheese, instant espresso, liquid sweetener and vanilla extract in blender and blend until combined well.

3. Now pour in coffee and gelatin mixture and blend until smooth.

4. Finally add whipping cream in mixture and blend on high until thick and whipped.

5. Pour mixture in serving cup and place in refrigerator for 2 hours then enjoy.

Nutritional Value per Serving

Protein: 8g   Fat: 16g   Carbs: 1.5g   Kcal: 175

Ketogenic Snack Recipes

Quick Cabbage Noodles

Time: 35 minutes   Servings: 2

Ingredients

- ¼ cup coconut oil
- 450g sliced green cabbage
- Salt

Directions

1. Preheat oven at 420F.

2. Line baking tray with foil.

3. Spared slice green cabbage on baking tray and drizzle some coconut oil and season with salt toss the cabbage well until cabbage is lightly coated with coconut oil.

4. Bake cabbage for 15 minutes after 15 minutes stir cabbage well and bake another 15 minutes again.

5. When cabbage look tender then stir and serve.

Nutritional Value per Serving

Protein: 3.5g   Fat: 9g   Carbs: 1g   Kcal: 85

Bun-Free Avocado Cheese Burger

Time: 25 minutes   Servings: 4

Ingredients

- 1 avocado

- 110g sliced yellow cheddar cheese

- 450g ground beef

- Salt

- Pepper

Directions

1. Take bowl and add ground beef then season with salt and pepper mix all well until combined after that make four burger patties.

2. Grill the patties until they cooked.

3. Then transfer cook patties in plate then lay quarter slice of avocado on each patty.

4. Then cover avocado with cheddar cheese slice.

5. Now use piece of foil to cover patties this will allow the residual heat to melt the cheese.

6. Once cheese is melted then serve burgers.

Nutritional Value per Serving

Protein: 29g   Fat: 33g   Carbs: 0.95g   Kcal: 405

Keto Stuffed Eggs

Time: 20 minutes   Servings: 6

Ingredients

- 6 boiled eggs
- 1 tbsp vinegar
- ½ tsp minced garlic
- ¾ tsp chili powder

- 1 tbsp minced onion
- 2 tbsp mayonnaise
- 1 tbsp yogurt

Directions

1. Peel the boiled eggs and sliced in half.

2. Remove the yolks carefully in bowl and arrange white in plate.

3. Mash yolk in bowl then add mayonnaise and yogurt stir well until mixture is smooth. Then add vinegar, garlic and onion and mix well until combined.

4. Now spoon the mixture in egg whites and sprinkle some chili powder on top and serve.

Nutritional Value per Serving

Protein: 3g   Fat: 9g   Carbs: 1g   Kcal: 85

Tuna and Cheese Stuffed Mushroom

Time: 30 minutes   Servings: 15

Ingredients

- 225g mushroom
- 1 spring onion, finely minced
- 3 tbsp mayonnaise

- 170g tuna
- 60g shredded Gouda cheese
- 2 tbsp grated parmesan cheese

Directions

1. Preheat the oven at 360F.

2. Then wipe mushroom clean with damp cloth and remove steams.

3. Now combined parmesan, Gouda, mayonnaise, tuna and spring onion and mix well until combined mixture.

4. Then spoon the mixture in mushroom cap arrange them in a baking pan. Add enough water to cover the bottom of pan.

5. Bake for 15 minutes and serve hot.

Nutritional Value per Serving

Protein: 5g   Fat: 7g   Carbs: 1g   Kcal: 55

Crunchy Smoked Almonds

Time: 45 minutes   Servings: 12

Ingredients

- 450g almonds
- 2 tsp BBQ rub
- 3 tbsp butter

- 2 tsp liquid smoke
- 2 tsp salt

Directions

1. Preheat the oven at 310F.

2. Place flat roasting pan over the burner and melt the butter in it. Stir seasoning into the butter.

3. Now add almonds in butter and mix well until well-coated.

4. Roast for 35 minutes and store in container.

Nutritional Value per Serving

Protein: 10g   Fat: 22g   Carbs: 3g   Kcal: 240   Fiber: 4g

Low-Carb Shrimp

Time: 120 minutes

Servings: 20

Ingredients

- 2kg shrimp

- 1 tbsp salt

- 350ml light beer

- 80g crab boils spices

Directions

1. Take slow cooker and add crab boil spices and light beer. Add salt and stir well.

2. Add shrimp in cooker and add enough water to bring liquid level up to top of the shrimp.

3. Now cover the cooker and set it to high and let it cook for 110 minutes.

4. Serve the shrimp straight from cooker with low-carb sauce.

Nutritional Value per Serving

Protein: 19g   Fat: 5g   Carbs: 1g   Kcal: 125

Cheese and Sunflower Crackers

Time: 40 minutes   Servings: 6

Ingredients

- 180g grated cheddar cheese
- 340g raw sunflower seeds

- ¼ cup water
- ½ tsp salt

Directions

1. Preheat the oven at 320F.

2. Add sunflower seed in food processor and grind to sunflower seed fine meal.

3. Now add cheddar cheese and salt and plus the processor 6 to 7 times. Then add water and plus until dough form.

4. Then roll the dough and make thinner sheet as you wanted then sprinkle some salt over the top.

5. Now use pizza cutter and cut square shape pieces and bake about 30 minutes and store crackers in airtight container.

Nutritional Value per Serving

Protein: 1g   Fat: 6g   Carbs: 0.5g   Kcal: 70   Fiber: 0.5g

Cream Cheese Spinach

Time: 20 minutes   Servings: 3

Ingredients

- 280g frozen spinach
- 25g parmesan cheese
- 120g heavy cream
- 2 tbsp butter
- Pepper and Salt

Directions

1. Cook spinach and drain very well squeeze out as much water as possible.

2. Then add drained spinach in bowl and add heavy cream, butter and cheese and stir well until cheese and butter completely melted.

3. Then season spinach with salt and pepper and serve immediately.

Nutritional Value per Serving

Protein: 6g   Fat: 19g   Carbs: 1.5g   Kcal: 190

Artichoke Cheese Dip

Time: 50 minutes   Servings: 4

Ingredients

- 380g artichoke hearts
- 110g grated parmesan cheese
- 1 garlic clove crushed
- 220g mayonnaise

Directions

1. Preheat the oven at 320F.

2. Then drain and chop in small pieces artichoke heart. Mix artichoke heart with garlic, cheese and mayonnaise and combined well.

3. Add mixture in small dish and sprinkle paprika on top. Bake about 45 minutes and serve with crackers.

Nutritional Value per Serving

Protein: 10g   Fat: 12g   Carbs: 2g   Kcal: 120

Easy Garlic and Cheese Stuffing Mushroom

Time: 40 minutes

Servings: 6

Ingredients

- 170g mushroom

- 2 tbsp crushed pork rinds

- 170g garlic and cheese spread

Directions

1. Preheat the oven at 350F. Wipe mushroom with dump cloth and remove steam. Divide cheese in mushroom caps.

3. Sprinkle pork rind crumbs each mushroom cap. Arrange mushroom cap in baking tray. Add just enough water to cover the bottom of pan.

4. Bake mushroom cap about 30 minute and serve hot.

Nutritional Value per Serving

Protein: 5g   Fat: 6g   Carbs: 1g   Kcal: 50

Conclusion

Finally, if you enjoyed this book, then I'd like to ask you for a favor, would you be kind enough to leave a review for this book on Amazon? It'd be greatly appreciated!

You can do so by typing this link into your browser:

→ bit.ly/KetoReview ←

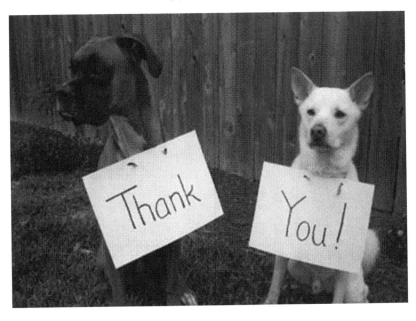

Thank you and good luck!

Free Bonus!

As you know, reading this book alone will not guarantee you any results. As with any goal, you must take action and stay motivated in the long term. For this reason, I've created an exclusive club for us to help each other on our ketogenic journeys, keep each other motivated and share each other's success. Together we can achieve the results we want!

I'm also giving away a FREE 30 Day Diet Plan Book with 90 of the tastiest Ketogenic Recipes for members only!

You can join The Ketogenic Dieters' Club for FREE by typing this link into your browser:

→ bit.ly/KetoClub ←

See you on the inside! – Oliver

41400933R00072

Made in the USA
San Bernardino, CA
11 November 2016